The inspiring Ketogenic Recipe Collection

Your guide to get in shape in the most rapid and healthy way

Martha McCarthy

2

TABLE OF CONTENTS

Eggplant Pizza with Tofu

Preparation Time: 15 minutes

Cooking Time: 45 minutes

Servings: 2

Ingredients:

- eggplants, sliced
- 1/3 cup butter, melted
- 2 garlic cloves, minced
- 1 red onion
- 12 oz tofu, chopped
- 7 oz tomato sauce
- Salt and black pepper to taste
- 1/2 tsp. cinnamon powder
- 1 cup Parmesan cheese, shredded
- 1/4 cup dried oregano

Directions:

1. Let the oven heat to 400F. Lay the eggplant slices on a baking sheet and brush with some butter. Bake in the oven until lightly browned, about 20 minutes.
2. Heat the remaining butter in a skillet; sauté garlic and onion until fragrant and soft, about 3 minutes.
3. Stir in the tofu and cook for 3 minutes. Add the tomato sauce, salt, and black pepper. Simmer for 10 minutes.

4. Sprinkle with the Parmesan cheese and oregano. Bake for 10 minutes.

Nutrition:

Calories: 321 Fat: 11.3g Fiber: 8.4g Carbohydrates: 4.3 g Protein: 10.1g

French Veggie Combo

Preparation Time: 52 minutes

Servings: 8

Ingredients:

- 3 cups cubed into ¼-inch pieces eggplant
- Salt, to taste
- 4 tbsp. olive oil -divided
- 1 chopped medium yellow onion
- 3 cups cubed into ¼-inch pieces zucchini
- minced garlic cloves
- 2 seeded and cubed into ½-inch pieces bell peppers
- 2 tbsp. thinly sliced basil leaves -divided
- ½ tsp red pepper flakes
- Freshly ground black pepper, to taste
- 2 cups cut into 1-inch pieces tomatoes
- 1 tbsp. chopped fresh parsley
- 1 tsp apple cider vinegar

Directions:

1. Arrange a colander in a sink.
2. Place eggplant pieces in the colander and sprinkle them with some salt. Keep aside to drain the moisture.
3. Place 2 tablespoons of the oil in the Instant Pot and select "Sauté." Then add the onion and cook for about 3-5 minutes.

4. Add the zucchini and garlic and cook for about 3-5 minutes.

5. Add the bell peppers and cook for about 3-5 minutes.

6. Add 1 tablespoon of basil leaves and stir to combine.

7. Select the "Cancel" and transfer the vegetable mixture to a bowl.

8. Place 2 tablespoons of the oil in the Instant Pot and select

9. "Sauté." Then add the drained eggplant and cook for about 3-4 minutes.

10. Select the "Cancel" and stir in a cooked veggie mixture of red pepper flakes and black pepper.

11. Arrange tomato slices on top.

12. Secure the lid and place the pressure valve in the "Seal" position.

13. Select "Manual" and cook under "High Pressure" for about 10 minutes.

14. Select the "Cancel" and carefully do a quick release.

15. Remove the lid and select "Sauté."

16. Stir in vinegar and cook for about 6- 8 minutes.

17. Select the "Cancel" and serve hot with the garnishing of the remaining basil.

Nutrition Values:

Calories 101, Total Fat 7.3g, Net Carbs 1.16g, Protein 1.8g, Fiber 2.9g

Gouda Cauliflower Casserole

Preparation Time: 15 minutes

Cooking Time: 15 minutes

Servings: 4

Ingredients:

- heads cauliflower, cut into florets
- 1/3 cup butter, cubed
- 2 tbsp. melted butter
- 1 white onion, chopped
- Salt and black pepper to taste
- 1/4 almond milk
- 1/2 cup almond flour
- 1/2 cups grated gouda cheese

Directions:

1. Preheat the oven to 350°F and put the cauliflower florets in a large microwave-safe bowl.
2. Sprinkle with a bit of water, and steam in the microwave for 4 to 5 minutes.
3. Melt the 1/3 cup of butter in a saucepan over medium heat and sauté the onion for 3 minutes.
4. Add the cauliflower, season with salt and black pepper, and mix in almond milk. Simmer for 3 minutes.
5. Mix the remaining melted butter with almond flour.

6. Stir into the cauliflower as well as half of the cheese. Sprinkle the top with the remaining cheese and bake for 10 minutes until the cheese has melted and golden brown.

7. Plate the bake and serve with salad.

Nutrition:

Calories: 349 Fat: 9.4g Fiber: 12.1g Carbohydrates: 4.1 g Protein: 10g

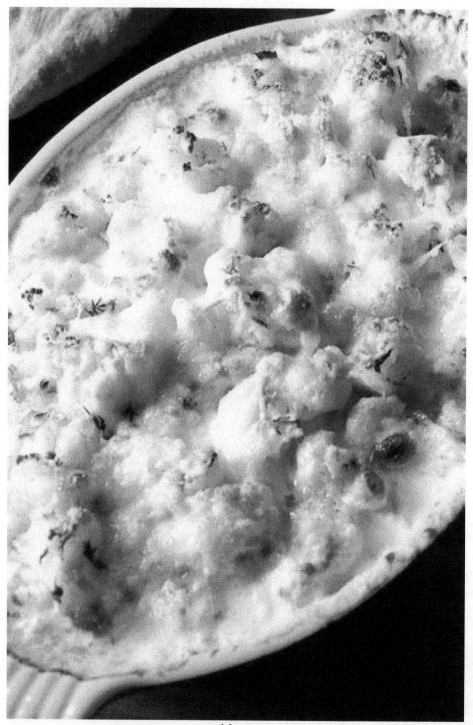

Indian Cabbage Stir-fry

Servings: 2

Cooking Time: 25 minutes

Ingredients

- 2 tablespoons olive oil
- 1 1-inch piece fresh ginger, grated
- 1/2 teaspoon cumin seeds
- 1 shallot, chopped
- 1/2 cup chicken stock
- 3/4 pound green cabbage, sliced
- 1/4 teaspoon turmeric powder
- 1/2 teaspoon coriander powder
- Kosher salt and cayenne pepper, to taste

Directions:

1. Heat the olive oil in a saucepan over medium heat; then, sauté the ginger and cumin seeds until fragrant.
2. Add in the shallot and continue sautéing an additional to 3 minutes or until just tender and aromatic. Pour in the chicken stock to deglaze the pan.
3. Add the cabbage wedges, turmeric, coriander, salt, and cayenne pepper.
4. Cover and cook for 15 to 18 minutes or until your cabbage has softened.

5. Make sure to stir occasionally.

6. Serve in individual bowls and enjoy!

Nutrition Info (Per Serving): 168 Calories; 13g Fat; 7g Total Carbs; 2.6g Protein; 4.1g Fiber

Indian Veggie Platter

Preparation Time: 22 minutes

Servings: 6

Ingredients:

- 4 dried red chilies
- 2 tbsp. shredded coconut
- 1 tsp coriander seeds
- 1 tsp cumin seeds
- ½ tsp mustard seeds
- ¼ tsp fenugreek seeds
- ½ tsp paprika
- 2 roughly chopped tomatoes
- ½ roughly chopped small yellow onion
- chopped garlic cloves
- Salt, to taste
- 2 tbsp. butter
- 3 cups cauliflower
- 3 cups green beans
- 1 cup seeded and chopped bell pepper
- 2 cups of water

Directions:

1. Heat a non-stick frying pan over medium heat and sauté red chilies, coconut, and spices for about 1-2 minutes.

2. Remove from heat and keep aside to cool slightly.

3. In a spice grinder, add the coconut mixture and grind it into a coarse powder.

4. In a blender, add the spice mixture, tomato, onion, garlic, and salt, and pulse until smooth.

5. Place the butter in the Instant Pot and select "Sauté." Then add the pureed tomato mixture and cook for about 4-5 minutes.

6. Select the "Cancel" and stir in veggies and water.

7. Secure the lid and place the pressure valve in the "Seal" position.

8. Select "Manual" and cook under "Low Pressure" for about 14-15 minutes.

9. Select the "Cancel" and carefully do a Natural release.

10. Remove the lid and serve.

Nutrition Values:

Calories 93, Total Fat 4.9g, Net Carbs 1.95g, Protein 3.1g, Fiber 4.4g

Keto Red Curry

Preparation Time: 20 minutes

Cooking Time: 15-20 minutes

Servings: 6

Ingredients:

- 1 cup broccoli florets
- 1 large handful of fresh spinach
- 4 Tbsp. coconut oil
- 1/4 medium onion
- 1 tsp. garlic, minced
- 1 tsp. fresh ginger, peeled and minced
- 2 tsp. soy sauce
- 1 Tbsp. red curry paste
- 1/2 cup coconut cream

Directions:

1. Add half the coconut oil to a saucepan and heat over medium-high heat.
2. When the oil is hot, put the onion in the pan and sauté for 3-4 minutes, until it is semi-translucent.
3. Sauté garlic, stirring, just until fragrant, about 30 seconds.
4. Lower the heat to medium-low and add broccoli florets. Sauté, stirring, for about 1-2 minutes.

5. Now, add the red curry paste. Sauté until the paste is fragrant, then mix everything.

6. Add the spinach on top of the vegetable mixture. When the spinach begins to wilt, add the coconut cream and stir.

7. Add the rest of the coconut oil, the soy sauce, and the minced ginger. Bring to a simmer for 5-10 minutes.

8. Serve hot.

Nutrition:

Calories: 265 Fat: 7.1g Fiber: 6.9g Carbohydrates: 2.1 g Protein: 4.4g

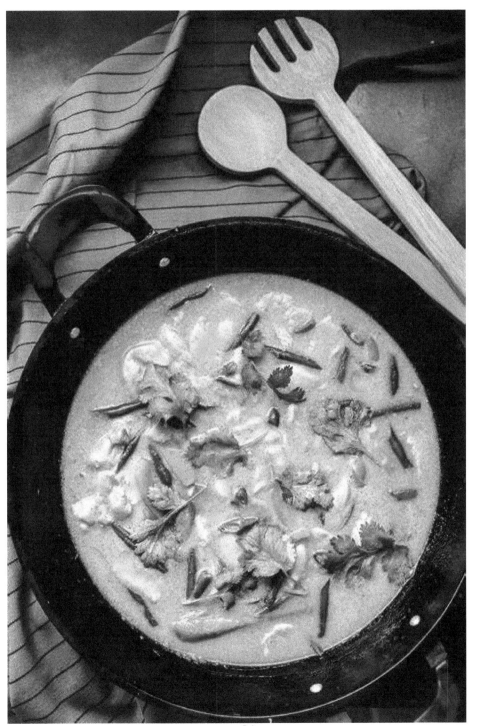

Lime Pork

Servings: 4

Cooking Time: 30 minutes

Ingredients

- 3 tablespoons olive oil
- 4 pork chops
- 1 cup beef stock
- A pinch of salt and black pepper
- 1 tablespoon lime juice
- 1 tablespoon lime zest, grated
- 2 tablespoons parsley, chopped

Directions:

1. Heat up a pan with the oil over medium-high heat, add the pork and brown for 5 minutes.
2. Add the stock and the other ingredients, toss, bring to a simmer and cook over medium heat for minutes more.
3. Divide everything between plates and serve.

Nutrition Info: calories 352, fat 30.5, fiber 0.2, carbs 0.4, protein 18.7

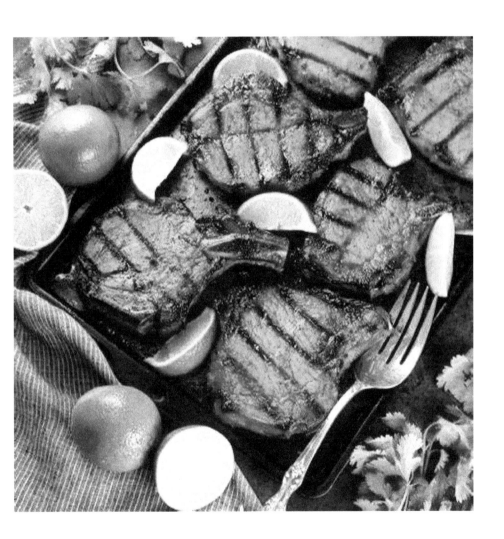

Mexican Casserole with Black Beans

Preparation Time: 20 minutes

Cooking Time: 20 minutes

Servings: 6

Ingredients:

- cups of minced garlic cloves
- 2 cups of Monterey Jack and cheddar
- 3/4 cup of salsa
- 1/2 cups chopped red pepper
- 2 teaspoons ground cumin
- cans black beans
- 12 corn tortillas
- 3 chopped tomatoes
- 1/2 cup of sliced black olives
- 2 cups of chopped onion

Directions:

1. Let the oven heat to 350° F.
2. Place a large pot over medium heat.
3. Pour the onion, garlic, pepper, cumin, salsa, and black beans in the pot —
4. Cook the ingredients for 3 minutes, stirring frequently. Arrange the tortillas in the baking dish.

5. Ensure they are well spaced and even overlapping the dish if necessary. Spread half of the bean's mixture on the tortillas. Sprinkle with the cheddar. Repeat the process across the tortillas until everything is well stuffed.

6. Cover the baking dish with foil paper and place in the oven.

7. Bake it for 15 minutes. Remove from the oven to cool down a bit. Garnish the casserole with olives and tomatoes.

Nutrition:

Calories: 325 Fat: 9.4g Fiber: 11.2g Carbohydrates: 3.1 g Protein: 12.6g

Mustard Greens Sauté

Servings: 4

Cooking Time: 20 minutes

Ingredients

- 1 tablespoon olive oil
- 1 pound mustard greens, roughly chopped
- 2 garlic cloves, minced
- 2 spring onions, chopped
- A pinch of salt and black pepper
- ½ cup chicken stock
- 1 tablespoon balsamic vinegar
- 1 tablespoon cilantro, chopped

Directions:

1. Heat up a pan with the oil over medium heat, add the garlic and the spring onions, stir and sauté for 5 minutes.
2. Add the mustard greens and the other ingredients, bring to a simmer and cook over medium heat for 15 minutes more. Divide everything between plates and serve.

Nutrition Info: calories 150, fat 12, fiber 2, carbs 4, protein 8

Old-fashioned Penuche Bars

Servings: 10

Cooking Time: 45 minutes

Ingredients

- 1/2 stick butter
- 2 tablespoons tahini sesame paste
- 1/2 cup almond butter
- 1 teaspoon Stevia
- 2 ounces baker's chocolate, sugar-free
- A pinch of salt
- A pinch of grated nutmeg
- 1/2 teaspoon cinnamon powder

Directions:

1. Microwave the butter for 30 to 35 seconds. Fold in the tahini, almond butter, Stevia, and chocolate.

2. Sprinkle with salt, nutmeg, and cinnamon; whisk to combine well. Scrape the mixture into a parchment-lined baking tray.

3. Transfer to the freezer for 40 minutes. Cut into bars and enjoy!

Nutrition Info (Per Serving): 176 Calories; 18.3g Fat; 3.2g Carbs; 1.8g Protein; 1.2g Fiber

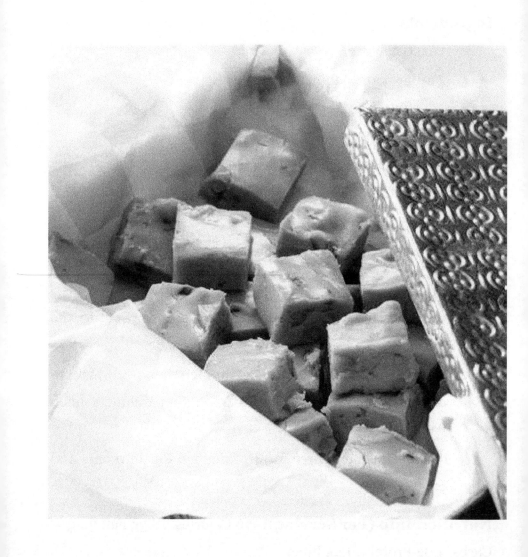

Seitan Kabobs with Bbq Sauce

Servings: 4

Cooking Time: 2 Hours 30 minutes

Ingredients

- 10 oz seitan, cut into chunks
- 1 ½ cups water
- 1 red onion, cut into chunks
- 1 red bell pepper, cut chunks
- 1 yellow bell pepper, chopped
- 2 tbsp olive oil
- 1 cup barbecue sauce
- Salt and black pepper to taste

Directions:

1. Bring the water to a boil into a pot, turn the heat off, and add seitan.
2. Cover the pot and let the tempeh steam for 5 minutes; drain.
3. Pour barbecue sauce into a bowl, add in the seitan, and coat with the sauce. Cover the bowl and then marinate in the fridge for 2 hours.
4. Preheat grill to 350° F, and thread the seitan, yellow bell pepper, red bell pepper, and onion. Brush the grate of the grill with some olive oil, place the skewers on it, and brush with barbecue sauce.

5. Cook the kabobs for 3 minutes on each side while rotating and brushing with more barbecue sauce. Serve.

Nutrition Info (Per Serving): Cal 228; Net Carbs 3.6g; Fat 15g; Protein 13.2g

South-East Asian Curry

Preparation Time: 42 minutes

Servings: 4

Ingredients:

- 3 cups sliced fresh mushrooms
- ½ tsp minced garlic
- Salt, to taste
- ¼ tsp ground coriander
- ¼ tsp ground cumin
- ¼ tsp ground turmeric
- ¼ tsp red chili powder
- ½ cup unsweetened coconut milk
- ¼ cup plain Greek yogurt

Directions:

1. In a Pyrex dish that will fit in an Instant Pot, add all ingredients and stir to combine.
2. In the bottom of the Instant Pot, arrange a steamer trivet and pour 1 cup of water.
3. Place the Pyrex dish on top of the trivet.
4. Secure the lid and place the pressure valve in the "Seal" position.

5. Select "Manual" and cook under "High Pressure" for about 27 minutes.

6. Select the "Cancel" and carefully do a "Natural" release.

7. Remove the lid and serve.

Nutrition Values:

Calories 93, Total Fat 7.6g, Net Carbs 2.22g, Protein 3.3g, Fiber 1.3g

Spicy Cauliflower Steaks with Steamed Green Beans

Preparation Time: 15 minutes

Cooking Time: 20 minutes

Servings: 4

Ingredients:

- heads cauliflower, sliced lengthwise into 'steaks.'
- 1/4 cup olive oil
- 1/4 cup chili sauce
- 2 tsp. erythritol
- Salt and black pepper to taste
- 2 shallots, diced
- 1 bunch green beans, trimmed
- 2 tbsp. fresh lemon juice
- 1 cup of water
- Dried parsley to garnish

Directions:

1. In a bowl or container, mix the olive oil, chili sauce, and erythritol. Brush the cauliflower with the mixture. Grill for 6 minutes. Flip the cauliflower, cook further for 6 minutes.

2. Let the water boil, place the green beans in a sieve, and set over the steam from the boiling water.

3. Cover with a clean napkin to keep the steam trapped in the sieve. Cook for 6 minutes.

4. After, remove to a bowl and toss with lemon juice.

5. Remove the grilled caulis to a plate; sprinkle with salt, pepper, shallots, and parsley. Serve with the steamed green beans.

Nutrition:

Calories: 329 Fat: 10.4g Fiber: 3.1g Carbohydrates: 4.2 g Protein: 8.4g

Spinach & Cucumber Tabbouleh

Servings: 6

Preparation Time: 10 minutes

Cooking Time: 5 minutes

Ingredients:

- Kanten Noodles: ½ oz.
- Carrots -julienned: 2
- Cauliflower rice: 3 cups
- Extra-virgin coconut oil: 2 tablespoon
- Salt: 1 teaspoon
- Cucumber -peeled, diced: 1
- Cherry tomatoes -chopped: 1 cup
- Spring onions -chopped: 2
- Spinach -chopped: 3 cups
- Parsley -chopped: 1 cup
- Mint -chopped: ½ cup
- Lemon juice: ½ cup
- Garlic clove -minced - 1
- Extra-virgin olive oil: ½ cup
- Ground black pepper: ¼ teaspoon

Directions:

1. Heat the coconut oil in a pan and cook the cauliflower rice for 5 minutes with a salt pinch. Set aside.

2. Whisk together the olive oil, garlic, and lemon juice.

3. Toss the cooked cauliflower rice with the rest of the ingredients, including the garlic sauce.

Nutrition Value:

245 Cal, 23.5 g total fat -5.6 g sat. fat, 8.4 g carb, 3 g fiber, 2.6 g protein.

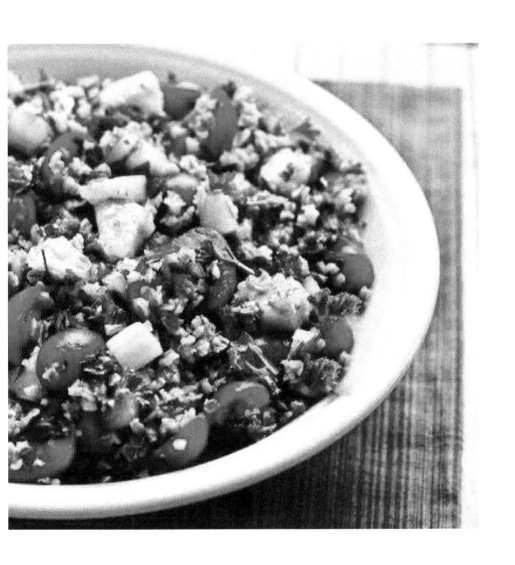

Stuffed Cremini Mushrooms

Servings: 4

Cooking Time: 35 minutes

Ingredients

- ½ head broccoli, cut into florets
- 1 pound cremini mushrooms, stems removed
- 2 tbsp coconut oil
- 1 onion, chopped
- 1 tsp garlic, minced
- 1 bell pepper, chopped
- 1 tsp cajun seasoning
- Salt and black pepper, to taste
- 1 cup cheddar cheese, shredded

Directions:

1. Use a food processor to pulse broccoli florets until they become small rice-like granules.

2. Set oven to 360°F. Bake mushroom caps until tender for 8 to 1minutes. In a heavy-bottomed skillet, melt the oil; stir in bell pepper, garlic, and onion and sauté until fragrant. Place in black pepper, salt, and cajun seasoning. Fold in broccoli rice.

3. Equally, separate the filling mixture among mushroom caps. Cover with cheddar cheese and bake for 17 more minutes. Serve warm.

Nutrition Info (Per Serving):

Kcal 206; Fat: 13.4g, Net Carbs: 10g, Protein: 12.7g

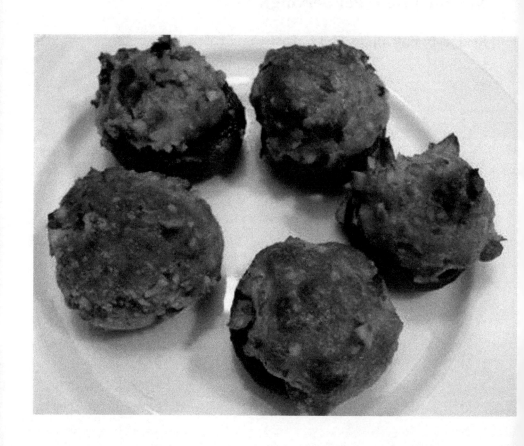

Summery Veggie Curry

Preparation Time: 29 minutes

Servings: 3

Ingredients:

For Spice Mixture:

- 1 tbsp. coriander seeds
- ½ tsp cumin seeds
- ½ tsp mustard seeds
- 2 tbsp. coconut shreds
- 2 tbsp. chopped peanuts
- 3 chopped garlic cloves
- 1 chopped hot green chile, chopped
- ½ tsp cayenne pepper
- ½ tsp ground turmeric
- Salt, to taste
- 1 tsp fresh lemon juice
- 1 cup plus 2 tsp water -divided
- baby eggplants

Directions:

1. Heat a non-stick frying pan over medium heat and sauté coriander, cumin, and mustard seeds for about 2 minutes.
2. Add the coconut and peanuts and sauté for about 1-2 minutes.
3. Remove from heat and keep aside to cool slightly.

4. In a small food processor, add coconut mixture, garlic, chile, spices, lemon juice, and 2 teaspoons of water and pulse until a coarse mixture is formed.

5. Carefully make cross cuts on each eggplant, not all the way through.

6. Fill the spice mixture into the crosscut.

7. In the pot of Instant Pot, place the eggplants and with 1 cup of water and ¼ teaspoon of salt.

8. Secure the lid and place the pressure valve in the "Seal" position.

9. Select "Manual" and cook under "High Pressure" for about 5 minutes.

10. Select the "Cancel" and carefully do a "Natural" release.

11. Remove the lid and serve.

Nutrition Values:

Calories 96, Total Fat 4.4g, Net Carbs 4.3g, Protein 4.1g, Fiber 5.1g

Sweet-And-Sour Tempeh

Preparation Time: 10 minutes

Cooking Time: 25 minutes

Servings: 4

Ingredients:

- Tempeh
- 1 package of tempeh
- 3/4 cup of vegetable broth
- 2 tablespoons of soy sauce
- 2 tablespoons olive oil Sauce
- can of pineapple juice
- tablespoons of brown sugar
- 1/4 cup of white vinegar
- 1 tablespoon of cornstarch
- 1 red bell pepper
- chopped white onion

Directions:

1. Place a skillet on high heat. Pour in the vegetable broth and tempeh in it.

2. Add the soy sauce to the tempeh. Let it cook until it softens. This usually takes 10 minutes.

3. When it is well cooked, remove the tempeh and keep the liquid. We are going to use it for the sauce.

4. Put the tempeh in another skillet placed on medium heat.

5. Sauté it with olive oil and cook until the tempeh is browned. This should take 3 minutes.

6. Place a pot of the reserved liquid from the cooked tempeh on medium heat.

7. Add the pineapple juice, vinegar, brown sugar, and cornstarch. Stir everything together until it's well combined.

8. Let it simmer for 5 minutes.

9. Add the onion and pepper to the sauce.

10. Stir in until the sauce is thick.

11. Reduce the heat, add the cooked tempeh and pineapple chunks to the sauce. Leave it to simmer together.

12. Remove from heat and serve with any grain food of your choice.

Nutrition:

Calories: 312 Fat: 10g Fiber: 4.1g Carbohydrates: 2.1 g Protein: 5.2g

Tofu Loaf with Walnuts

Servings: 4

Cooking Time: 70 minutes

Ingredients

- 3 tbsp olive oil
- 2 white onions, chopped
- 4 garlic cloves, minced
- 1 lb tofu, pressed and cubed
- 2 tbsp soy sauce
- ¾ cup chopped walnuts
- Salt and black pepper
- 1 tbsp Italian mixed herbs
- ½ tsp swerve sugar
- ¼ cup golden flaxseed meal
- 1 tbsp sesame seeds
- 1 green bell pepper, chopped
- 1 red bell pepper, chopped
- ½ cup tomato sauce

Directions:

1. Now, preheat the oven to 350F; then combine olive oil, onion, garlic, tofu, soy sauce, walnuts, salt, pepper, Italian herbs, swerve sugar, golden flaxseed meal and mix with your hands.

45

2. Pour the mixture into a bowl, stir in sesame seeds and bell peppers.

3. Transfer the loaf into a greased and spoon tomato sauce on top.

4. Bake for 45 minutes.

5. Turn onto a chopping board, slice, and serve.

Nutrition Info (Per Serving): Cal 432; Net Carbs 2.5g; Fat 31g; Protein 24g

Tofu Pops

Servings: 4

Cooking Time: 1 Hour 17 minutes

Ingredients

- 1 (14 oz) block tofu, cubed
- 1 bunch of chives, chopped
- 1 lemon, zested and juiced
- 12 slices bacon
- 12 mini skewers
- 1 tsp butter

Directions:

1. Mix chives, lemon zest, and juice in a bowl and toss the tofu cubes in the mixture. Marinate for an hour. Remove the zest and chives off the cubes and wrap each tofu in a bacon slice; insert each skewer and the bacon's end. Melt butter in a skillet and fry tofu skewers until the bacon browns and crisps. Serve with mayo dipping sauce.

Nutrition Info (Per Serving): Cal 392; Net Carbs 9g, Fat 22g, Protein 18g

Tofu Skillet with Vegetables & Avocado

Servings: 2

Cooking Time: 15 minutes

Ingredients

- 2 teaspoons olive oil
- 6 ounces firm tofu, pressed and cubed
- 4 tablespoons scallions, chopped
- 1 teaspoon ginger-garlic paste
- 2 cups enoki mushrooms
- 1 red bell pepper, sliced
- 1/2 teaspoon paprika
- Sea salt and ground black pepper, to taste
- 1/2 avocado, pitted, peeled and sliced

Directions:

1. Heat a teaspoon of olive oil in a nonstick skillet over a moderate flame. Now, fry the tofu cubes for 3 to 4 minutes, stirring to ensure even cooking; reserve.

2. In the same skillet, heat the remaining teaspoon of olive oil. Now, sauté the scallions for 3 minutes or until tender and fragrant.

3. Add in the ginger-garlic paste, mushrooms, and pepper; continue to sauté for minutes more or until tender.

4. Sprinkle the sautéed vegetables with the paprika, salt, and black pepper. Top with the reserved tofu. Serve with avocado. Devour!

Nutrition Info (Per Serving):

217 Calories; 17g Fat; 7.5g Carbs; 11.5g Protein; 4.5g Fiber

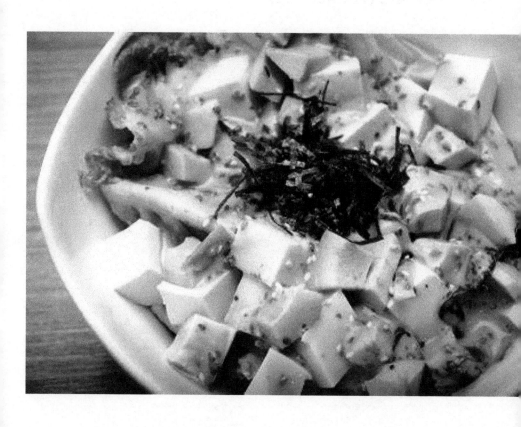

Tofu Skewers with Sesame Sauce

Servings: 4

Cooking Time: 15 minutes

Ingredients

- 2 tbsp tahini
- 1 (14 oz) firm tofu, cubed
- 1 zucchini, cut into wedges
- ¼ cup cherry tomatoes halved
- 1 red onion, cut into wedges
- 1 tbsp soy sauce
- 1 tbsp olive oil
- Sesame seeds for garnishing

Directions:

1. In a bowl, mix tahini and soy sauce; mix toss tofu in the sauce.
2. Let rest for 30 minutes. Thread tofu, zucchini, tomatoes and onion, alternately, on wooden skewers.
3. Heat olive oil in a grill pan then cooks tofu until golden brown, 8 minutes.
4. Serve garnished with sesame seeds.

Nutrition Info (Per Serving): Cal 266; Net Carbs 2.4g; Fat 19g; Protein 14g

Two-cheese Zucchini Gratin

Servings: 5

Cooking Time: 50 minutes

Ingredients

- 10 large eggs
- 3 tablespoons yogurt
- 2 zucchini, sliced
- 1/2 medium-sized leek, sliced
- Sea salt and ground black pepper, to taste
- 1 teaspoon cayenne pepper
- 1 cup cream cheese
- 2 garlic cloves, minced
- 1 cup Swiss cheese, shredded

Directions:

1. Start by preheating your oven to 360 degrees F. Then, spritz the bottom and sides of an ovenproof pan with a nonstick cooking spray. Then, mix the eggs with yogurt until well combined.

2. Overlap 1/2 of the zucchini and leek slices in the pan. Season with salt, black pepper, and cayenne pepper. Add cream cheese and minced garlic.

3. Add the remaining zucchini slices and leek. Add the egg mixture. Top with Swiss cheese. Bake for minutes until the top is golden brown. Bon appétit!

Nutrition Info (Per Serving): 371 Calories; 32g Fat; 5.2g Carbs; 0.3g Fiber; 15.7g Protein;

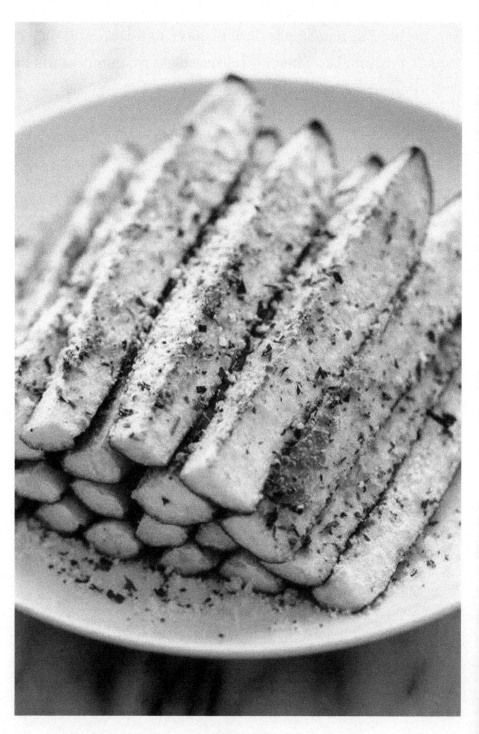

Vegetable Patties

Preparation Time: 15 minutes

Cooking Time: 20 minutes

Servings: 4

Ingredients:

- 1 tbsp. olive oil 1 onion, chopped
- 1 garlic clove, minced
- 1/2 head cauliflower, grated
- 1 carrot, shredded
- 3 tbsp. coconut flour
- 1/2 cup Gruyere cheese, shredded
- 1/2 cup Parmesan cheese, grated
- 2 eggs, beaten
- 1/2 tsp. dried rosemary
- Salt and black pepper, to taste

Directions:

1. Cook onion and garlic in warm olive oil over medium heat, until soft, for about 3 minutes.
2. Stir in grated cauliflower and carrot and cook for a minute; allow cooling and set aside.
3. To the cooled vegetables, add the rest of the ingredients, form balls from the mixture, then press each ball to form a burger patty.

4. Set oven to 400 F and bake the burgers for 20 minutes.

5. Flip and bake for another 10 minutes or until the top becomes golden brown.

Nutrition:

Calories: 315 Fat: 12.1g Fiber: 8.6g Carbohydrates: 3.3 g Protein: 5.8g

Veggie Greek Moussaka

Preparation Time: 20 minutes

Cooking Time: 30 minutes

Servings: 6

Ingredients:

- large eggplants, cut into strips
- 1 cup diced celery
- 1 cup diced carrots
- 1 small white onion, chopped
- 2 eggs
- 1 tsp. olive oil
- 3 cups grated Parmesan
- 1 cup ricotta cheese
- 3 cloves garlic, minced
- 2 tsp. Italian seasoning blend
- Salt to taste

Sauce:

- 1 1/2 cups heavy cream
- 1/4 cup butter, melted
- cup grated mozzarella cheese
- 2 tsp. Italian seasoning
- 3/4 cup almond flour

Directions:

1. Preheat the oven to 350º F.

2. Lay the eggplant strips, sprinkle with salt, and let sit there to exude liquid. Heat olive oil heat and sauté the onion, celery, garlic, and carrots for 5 minutes.

3. Mix the eggs, 1 cup of Parmesan cheese, ricotta cheese, and salt in a bowl; set aside.

4. Pour the heavy cream into a pot and bring to heat over a medium fire while continually stirring.

5. Stir in the remaining Parmesan cheese and one teaspoon of Italian seasoning. Turn the heat off and set it aside.

6. To lay the moussaka, spread a small amount of the sauce at the baking dish's bottom.

7. Pat dry the eggplant strips and make a single layer on the sauce.

8. A layer of ricotta cheese must be spread on the eggplants, sprinkle some veggies on it, and repeat everything

9. Evenly mix the melted butter, almond flour, and one teaspoon of Italian seasoning in a small bowl.

10. Spread the top of the moussaka layers with it and sprinkle the top with mozzarella cheese.

11. Bake for 25 minutes until the cheese is slightly burned. Slice the moussaka and serve warm.

Nutrition:

Calories: 398 Fat: 15.1g Fiber: 11.3g Carbohydrates: 3.1 g Protein: 5.9g

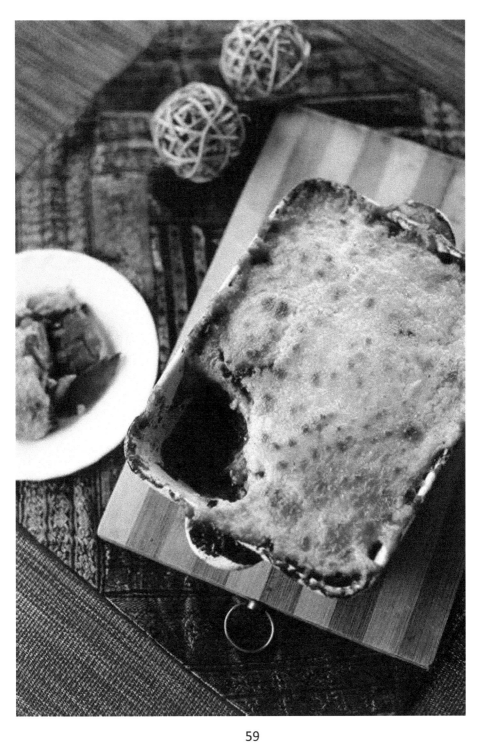

Almond Butter Fat Bombs

Servings: 4

Cooking Time: 3 minutes + Cooling Time

Ingredients

- ½ cup almond butter
- ½ cup of coconut oil
- 4 tbsp unsweetened cocoa powder
- ½ cup erythritol

Directions:

1. Melt butter and coconut oil in the microwave for 45 seconds, stirring twice until properly melted and mixed.

2. Mix in cocoa powder and erythritol until completely combined.

3. Pour into muffin moulds and refrigerate for 3 hours to harden.

Nutrition Info (Per Serving): Kcal 193, Fat 18.3g, Net Carbs 2g, Protein 4g

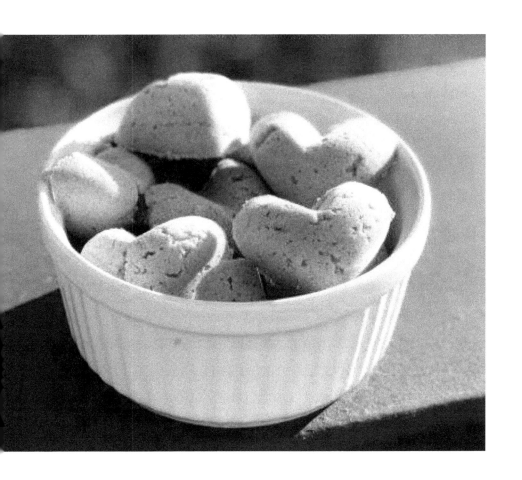

Bacon Braised Cabbage

Servings: 2

Cooking Time: 10 minutes

Ingredients

- 4 strips of bacon, sliced
- 1 cup sliced cabbage
- 1 tsp avocado oil
- 2 tbsp water

Seasoning:

- 1/3 tsp salt
- 1/4 tsp ground black pepper

Directions:

1. Take a skillet pan, place it over medium heat and when hot, add bacon pieces and cook for 4 to 5 minutes until browned on all sides.

2. Add cabbage, stir in water and then cook for 4 to 5 minutes until the cabbage has turned soft. Drizzle with oil, season with salt and black pepper, continue cooking for 2 minutes and then Serve.

Nutrition Info: 150 Calories; 10.7 g Fats; 9.1 g Protein; 2.1 g Net Carb; 1.2 g Fiber

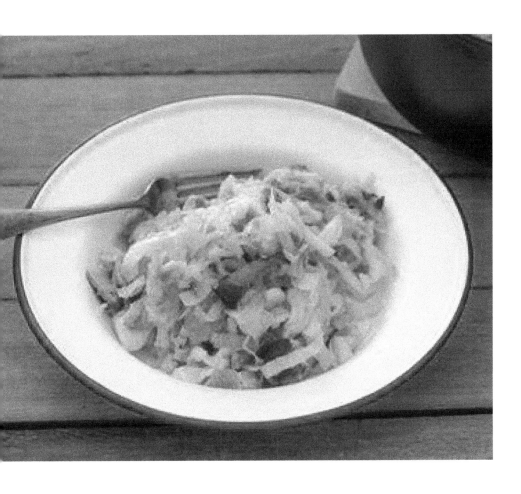

Bacon & Cheese Zucchini Balls

Servings: 6

Cooking Time: 3 Hours 20 minutes

Ingredients

- 4 cups zoodles
- ½ pound bacon, chopped
- 6 ounces cottage cheese, curds
- 6 ounces cream cheese
- 1 cup fontina cheese
- ½ cup dill pickles, chopped, squeezed
- 2 cloves garlic, crushed
- 1 cup grated Parmesan cheese
- ½ tsp caraway seeds
- ¼ tsp dried dill weed
- ½ tsp onion powder
- Salt and black pepper, to taste
- 1 cup crushed pork rinds
- Cooking oil

Directions:

1. Thoroughly mix zoodles, cottage cheese, dill pickles, ½ cup of Parmesan cheese, garlic, cream cheese, bacon, and fontina cheese until well combined. Shape the mixture into balls. Refrigerate for 3 hours.

2. In a mixing bowl, mix the remaining ½ cup of Parmesan cheese, crushed pork rinds, dill, black pepper, onion powder, caraway seeds, and salt. Roll cheese ball in Parmesan mixture to coat.

3. Set a skillet over medium heat, then warm 1-inch of oil. Fry cheese balls until browned on all sides. Set on a paper towel.

Nutrition Info (Per Serving): Kcal 407; Fat: 26.8g, Net Carbs: 5.8g, Protein: 33.4g

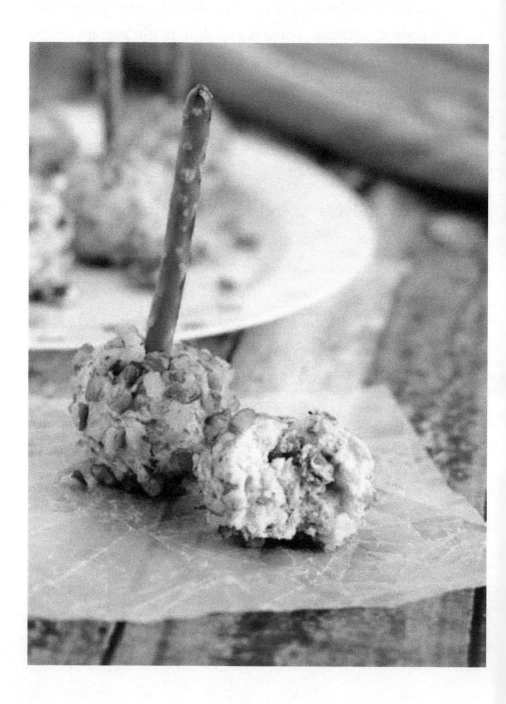

Baked Zucchini Gratin

Preparation Time: 25 minutes

Cooking Time: 30 minutes

Servings: 2

Ingredients:

- large zucchini, cut into 1/4-inch-thick slices
- Pink Himalayan salt
- 1-ounce Brie cheese, rind trimmed off
- 1 tablespoon butter
- Freshly ground black pepper
- 1/3 cup shredded Gruyere cheese
- 1/4 cup crushed pork rinds

Directions:

1. Preheat the oven to 400° F.
2. When the zucchini has been "Weeping" for about 30 minutes, in a small saucepan over medium-low heat, heat the Brie and butter, occasionally stirring, until the cheese has melted.
3. The mixture is thoroughly combined for about 2 minutes.
4. Arrange the zucchini in an 8-inch baking dish, so the zucchini slices are overlapping a bit.
5. Season with pepper.

6. Pour the Brie mixture over the zucchini, and top with the shredded Gruyere cheese.

7. Sprinkle the crushed pork rinds over the top.

8. Bake for about 25 minutes, until the dish is bubbling and the top is nicely browned, and serve.

Nutrition:

Calories: 324 Fat: 11.5g Fiber: 5.1g Carbohydrates: 2.2 g Protein: 5.1g

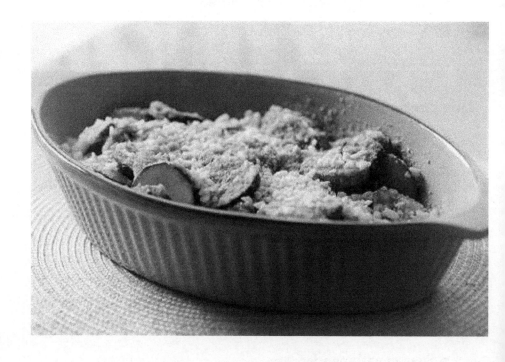

Basil Turkey Meatballs

Servings: 4

Cooking Time: 15 minutes

Ingredients

- 1 pound ground turkey
- 2 tbsp chopped sun-dried tomatoes
- 2 tbsp chopped basil
- ½ tsp garlic powder
- 1 egg
- ½ tsp salt
- ¼ cup almond flour
- 2 tbsp olive oil
- ½ cup shredded mozzarella cheese
- ¼ tsp pepper

Directions:

1. Place everything except the oil in a bowl. Mix with your hands until combined.
2. Form into balls. Heat the olive oil in a skillet over medium heat.
3. Cook the meatballs for 4-5 minutes per each side. Serve.

Nutrition Info (Per Serving): Kcal 310, Fat: 26g, Net Carbs: 2g, Protein: 22g

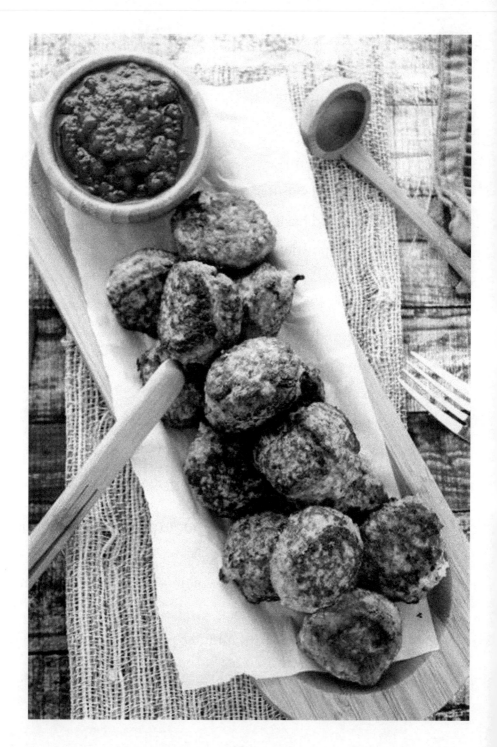

Bell Pepper & Pumpkin with Avocado Sauce

Servings: 4

Cooking Time: 15 minutes

Ingredients

- ½ pound pumpkin, peeled
- ½ pound bell peppers
- 1 tbsp olive oil
- 1 avocado, peeled and pitted
- 1 lemon, juiced and zested
- 2 tbsp sesame oil
- 2 tbsp cilantro, chopped
- 1 onion, chopped
- 1 jalapeño pepper, deveined and minced
- Salt and black pepper, to taste

Directions:

1. Use a spiralizer to spiralize bell peppers and pumpkin. Using a large nonstick skillet, warm olive oil.

2. Add in bell peppers and pumpkin and sauté for 8 minutes. Combine the remaining ingredients to obtain a creamy mixture. Top the vegetable noodles with the avocado sauce and serve.

Nutrition Info (Per Serving): Kcal 233; Fat: 20.2g, Net Carbs: 11g, Protein: 1.9g

Black Bean Veggie Burger

Preparation Time: 15 minutes

Cooking Time: 20 minutes

Servings: 2

Ingredients:

- 1/2 onion (chopped small)
- 1 (14-ounce) can of black beans (well-drained)
- 2 slices of bread (crumbled)
- 1/2 teaspoon of seasoned salt
- 1 teaspoon of garlic powder
- 1 teaspoon of onion powder
- 1/2 cup of almond flour
- Dash salt (to taste)
- Dash pepper (to taste)
- Oil for frying (divide)

Directions:

1. Combine onions and sauté and pour it into the small frying pan. Fry them until they are soft. This process usually takes between 3 and 5 minutes.
2. Get a large bowl. Mash the black beans inside it. Ensure that the beans are almost smooth.
3. Sauté your onions and crumble the bread.

4. In the bowl, add the sautéed onions, mashed black beans, crumbled bread, seasoned salt, garlic powder, and onion powder. Ensure you mix to combine well.

5. Add some flour to the ingredients by adding a teaspoon per time. Stir everything together until it is well combined.

6. While mixing, make sure that it is very thick.

7. To achieve this, you may want to use your hand to work your flour well. Make the mixed black beans into patties.

8. Ensure that each of the patties is approximately 1/2 inch thick.

9. The best way to do this is to make a ball with the black beans.

10. After doing this, flatten the ball gently. Place your frying pan on medium-low heat. Add some oil.

11. Fry your black bean patties in the frying pan until it is slightly firm and lightly browned on each side. This usually takes about 3 minutes.

12. Ensure you adjust the head well because if the pan is too hot, the bean burgers will be brown in the middle and will not be well cooked in the middle.

13. To serve, assemble your veggie burgers and enjoy them with all the fixings. You can also serve to get a plate, serve them with a little ketchup or hot sauce. To increase the nutrition of the meal, you can add a nice green salad.

Nutrition: Calories: 376 Fat: 15.1g Fiber: 12.9g Carbohydrates: 9.4 g Protein: 11.6g

Broccoli and Bacon Stir-fry

Servings: 2

Cooking Time: 15 minutes

Ingredients

- 6-oz broccoli florets, chopped
- 4 oz ground turkey
- 2 green onions, chopped
- 2 slices of bacon, cooked, crumbled
- ¼ tsp dried thyme Seasoning:
- ½ tsp salt
- ¼ tsp ground black pepper

Directions:

1. Take a skillet pan, place it over medium heat, add bacon slices, and cook for 5 minutes until crispy.
2. Transfer bacon to a cutting board, cool for 5 minutes, then crumble it and set aside until required.
3. Add turkey into the pan, cook for 3 minutes until turkey is no longer pink, then add broccoli and onions, season with salt, black pepper, and thyme, stir well and continue cooking for 5 to 7 minutes until thoroughly cooked.
4. When done, top with bacon and serve.

Nutrition Info: 481 Calories; 38 g Fats; 30 g Protein; 2.7 g Net Carb; 2.1 g Fiber;

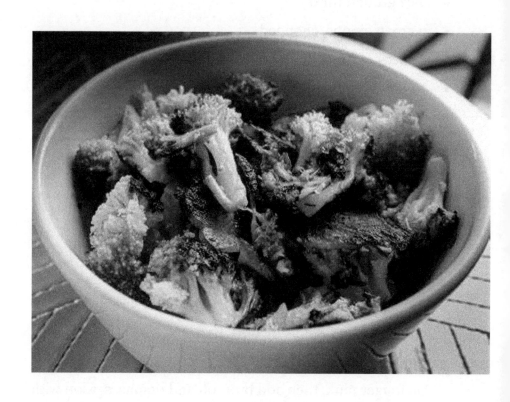

Broccoli and Cheddar Fritters

Servings: 2

Cooking Time: 8 minutes

Ingredients

- 2 slices of bacon, chopped, cooked
- 4 oz broccoli florets, chopped
- 1 tbsp coconut flour
- 2 oz grated cheddar cheese
- 1 egg

Seasoning:

- ½ tsp Cajun seasoning
- 1 tbsp avocado oil

Directions:

1. Take a medium heatproof bowl, place broccoli florets in it, drizzle with tbsp water, cover the bowl with a plastic wrap, and then microwave for 2 to 3 minutes at a high heat setting until tender.
2. Drain the broccoli, pat dry with paper towels, then transfer broccoli into a bowl and stir in flour and Cajun seasoning until mixed.
3. Add egg and cheddar cheese and then stir until well combined.

4. Take a medium skillet pan, place it over medium heat, add oil and when hot, spoon broccoli mixture in it in the form of mounds and then cook for 2 to 3 minutes per side until golden brown. Serve.

Nutrition Info:

303 Calories; 22.7 g Fats; 16.3 g Protein; 4.1 g Net Carb; 2.6 g Fiber;

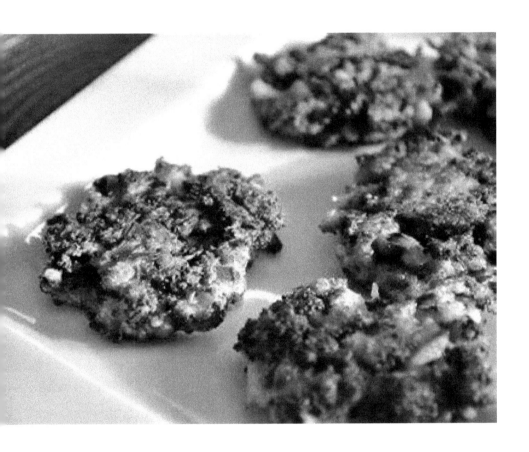

Broccoli, Green Beans and Bacon Stir-fry

Servings: 2

Cooking Time: 13 minutes

Ingredients

- 4 oz broccoli florets
- 2 oz green beans
- 4 slices of bacon, cooked, crumbled
- 1 tbsp chopped parsley
- 1 tbsp coconut oil

Seasoning:

- ½ tsp salt
- 1/8 tsp ground black pepper

Directions:

1. Take a skillet pan, place it over medium heat, add bacon, and cook for 5 minutes until crispy. Then transfer bacon to a cutting board, let it cool for 5 minutes, then crumble it and set aside until required.

2. Add broccoli and beans into the pan, add oil, season with salt and black pepper and cook for 5 to 7 minutes or until tender. Return bacon into the pan, stir well, cook for a minute and then remove the pan from heat. Garnish with parsley and serve.

Nutrition Info: 522 Calories; 47 g Fats; 22.2 g Protein; 0.5 g Net Carb; 2.1 g Fiber;

Brussel Sprouts with Spiced Halloumi

Preparation Time: 20 minutes

Cooking Time: 30 minutes

Servings: 2

Ingredients:

- 10 oz halloumi cheese, sliced
- 1 tbsp. coconut oil
- 1/2 cup unsweetened coconut, shredded
- 1 tsp. chili powder
- 1/2 tsp. onion powder
- 1/2 pound Brussels sprouts, shredded
- 4 oz butter
- Salt and black pepper to taste
- Lemon wedges for serving

Directions:

1. In a bowl, mix the shredded coconut, chili powder, salt, coconut oil, and onion powder.
2. Then, toss the halloumi slices in the spice mixture.
3. The grill pan must be heated, then cook the coated halloumi cheese for 2-3 minutes.
4. Transfer to a plate to keep warm.

5. The half butter must be melted in a pan, add, and sauté the Brussels sprouts until slightly caramelized.

6. Then, season with salt and black pepper.

7. Dish the Brussels sprouts into serving plates with the halloumi cheese and lemon wedges.

8. Melt left butter and drizzle over the Brussels sprouts and halloumi cheese. Serve.

Nutrition:

Calories: 276 Fat: 9.5g Fiber: 9.1g Carbohydrates: 4.1 g Protein: 5.4g

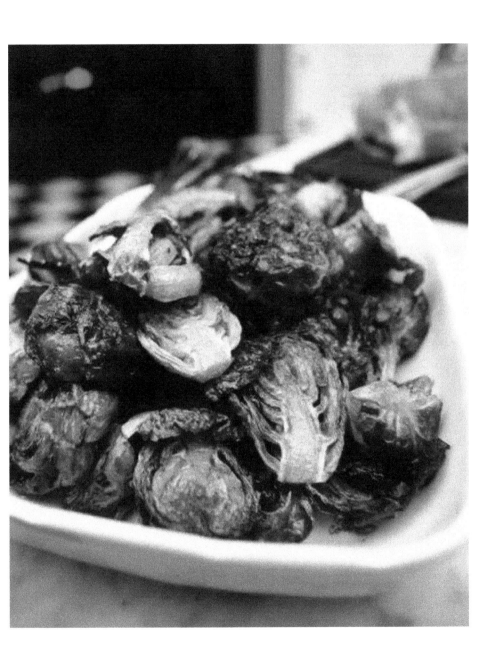

Celery Boats with Gruyère Cheese

Servings: 2

Cooking Time: 35 minutes

Ingredients

- 1 jalapeno pepper, deveined and minced
- 1/4 teaspoon sea salt
- 1/4 teaspoon ground black pepper
- 1 teaspoon granulated garlic
- 3 tablespoons scallions, minced
- 1/2 teaspoon caraway seeds
- 2 ounces Gruyère cheese
- 3 celery stalks, halved

Directions:

1. In a mixing bowl, thoroughly combine the minced jalapeno with sea salt, black pepper, garlic, scallions, caraway seeds, and Gruyère cheese. Spread this mixture over the celery stalks. Then, arrange them on a parchment-lined baking tray.

2. Roast in the preheated oven at 0 degrees F for 35 minutes or until cooked through.

Nutrition Info (Per Serving): 194 Calories; 17.1g Fat; 7g Carbs; 2.5g Protein; 5g Fiber

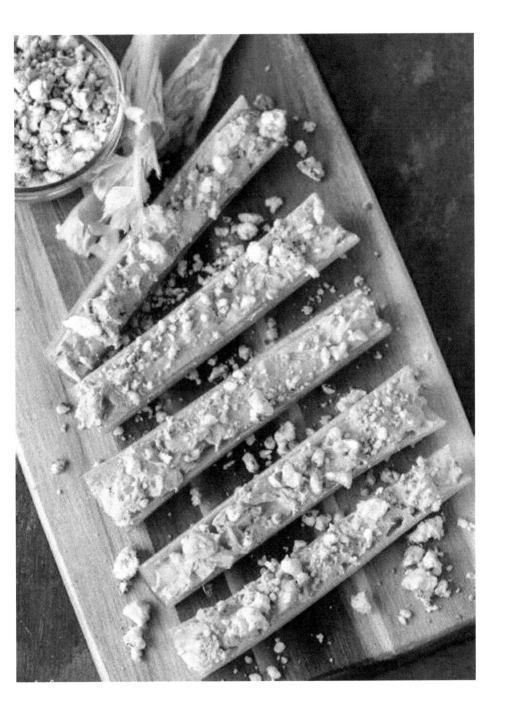

Cheddar Cauliflower Bites

Servings: 8

Cooking Time: 25 minutes

Ingredients

- 1 pound cauliflower florets
- 1 teaspoon sweet paprika
- A pinch of salt and black pepper
- 2 eggs, whisked
- 1 cup coconut flour
- Cooking spray
- 1 cup cheddar cheese, grated

Directions:

1. In a bowl, mix the flour with salt, pepper, cheese and paprika and stir.
2. Put the eggs in a separate bowl.
3. Dredge the cauliflower florets in the eggs and then in the cheese mix, arrange them on a baking sheet lined with parchment paper and bake at 0 degrees F for 25 minutes.
4. Serve as a snack.

Nutrition Info: calories 163, fat 12, fiber 2, carbs 2, protein 7

Cheese Scallops with Chorizo

Servings: 4

Cooking Time: 15 minutes

Ingredients

- 2 tbsp ghee
- 16 fresh scallops
- 8 ounces chorizo, chopped
- 1 red bell pepper, sliced
- 1 cup red onions, chopped
- 1 cup Parmesan, grated

Directions:

1. Melt half of the ghee in a skillet and cook onion and bell pepper for 5 minutes.
2. Add in chorizo and stir-fry for another 3 minutes; set aside.
3. Season scallops with salt and pepper.
4. Add all the remaining ghee to the skillet and sear the scallops for 2 minutes on each side.
5. Add the chorizo mixture back and warm through.
6. Transfer to Serves platter and top with Parmesan cheese to serve.

Nutrition Info (Per Serving): Cal 491; Net Carbs 5g; Fat 32g; Protein 36g

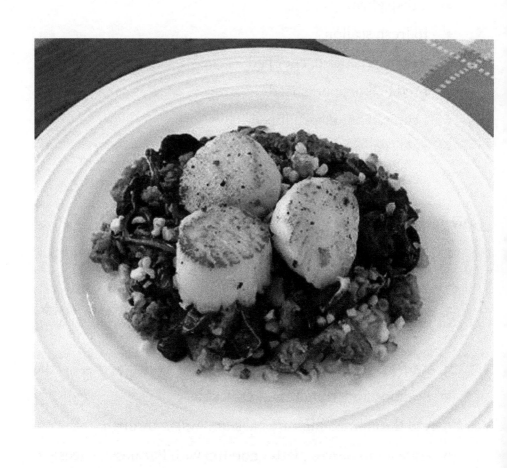

Cheesy Cauliflower Falafel

Preparation Time: 20 minutes

Cooking Time: 15 minutes

Servings: 4

Ingredients:

- 1 head cauliflower, cut into florets
- 1/3 cup silvered ground almonds
- 2 tbsp. cheddar cheese, shredded
- 1/2 tsp. mixed spice
- Salt and chili pepper to taste
- 3 tbsp. coconut flour
- fresh eggs
- tbsp. ghee

Directions:

1. Blend the florets in a blender until a grain meal consistency is formed.
2. Pour the rice into a bowl, add the ground almonds, mixed spice, salt, cheddar cheese, chili pepper, coconut flour, and mix until evenly combined.
3. Beat the eggs in a bowl until creamy in color and mix with the cauliflower mixture.
4. Shape 1/4 cup each into patties.

5. Melt ghee and fry the patties for 5 minutes on each side to be firm and browned.

6. Remove onto a wire rack to cool, share into serving plates, and top with tahini sauce.

Nutrition:

Calories: 287 Fat: 9.2g Fiber: 4.1g Carbohydrates: 3.2 g Protein: 13.2g

Cheesy Spinach-Egg Bake

Servings: 4

Preparation Time: 10 minutes

Cooking Time: 35 minutes

Ingredients:

- Eggs - 6
- Fresh baby spinach: 5 oz.
- Mozzarella cheese -shredded: 6 oz.
- Heavy cream: 1/3 cup
- Butter: 1 tablespoon
- Green onions -sliced thinly: ½ oz.
- Salt: ½ teaspoon
- Pepper: ½ teaspoon

Directions:

1. Whisk together the egg, cream, salt, and pepper.
2. Melt butter in a pan and sauté the spinach in it until wilted.
3. Place the spinach in a baking dish greased with a non-stick spray.
4. Sprinkle the Mozzarella cheese and the green onions.
5. Pour the egg over, gently stirring.
6. Bake in an oven preheated to 375 degrees Fahrenheit for 35 minutes.

Nutrition Value:

339 Cal, 24 g total fat, 2 g carbs, 22 g protein.

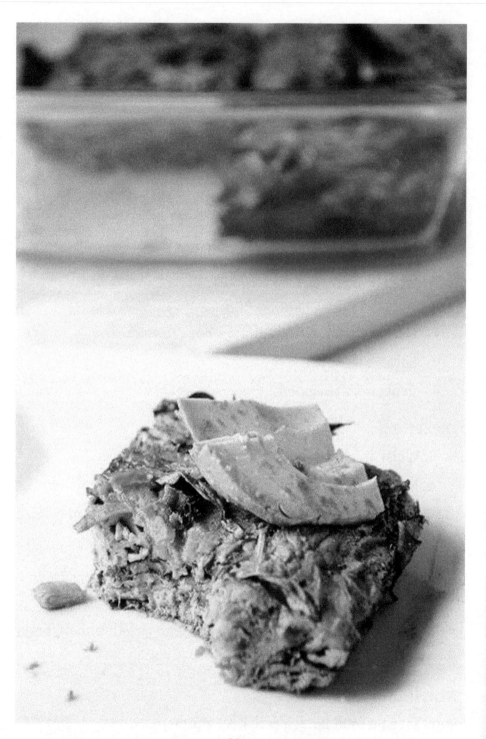

Cherry Tomato Salad with Chorizo

Servings: 4

Cooking Time: 10 minutes

Ingredients

- 2 ½ cups cherry tomatoes
- 2 ½ tbsp olive oil
- 4 chorizo sausages, chopped
- 2 tsp red wine vinegar
- 1 small red onion, chopped
- 2 tbsp chopped cilantro
- Salt and black pepper to taste
- Sliced Kalamata olives

Directions:

1. Heat tbsp of olive oil into a skillet and fry the chorizo until golden.
2. Cut in half tomatoes.
3. In a salad bowl, whisk the remaining olive oil with vinegar and add onion, tomatoes, cilantro, and chorizo.
4. Mix to coat in the dressing; season with salt and pepper.
5. Garnish with olives to serve.

Nutrition Info (Per Serving): Cal 138; Net Carbs 5.2g; Fat 8.9g; Protein 7g

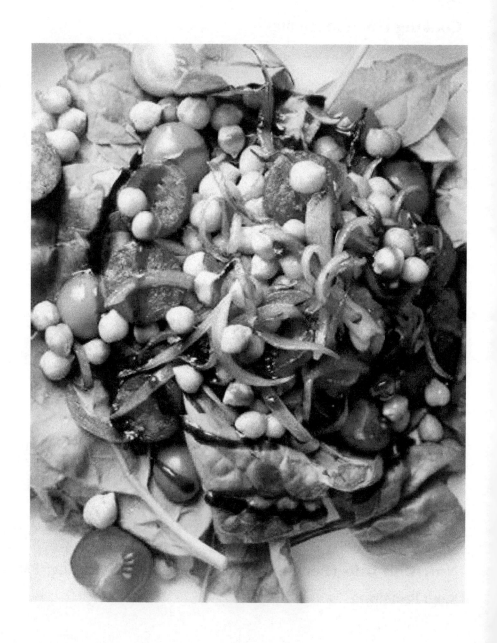

Chili Beef Stew with Cauliflower Grits

Servings: 4

Cooking Time: 55 minutes

Ingredients

- 2 tbsp olive oil
- 2 lb chuck roast, cubed
- 1 large yellow onion, chopped
- 3 garlic cloves, minced
- 2 large tomatoes, diced
- 1 tbsp rosemary
- 1 tbsp smoked paprika
- 2 tsp chili powder
- 2 cups beef broth
- 2 tbsp butter
- ½ cup walnuts, chopped
- 2 cups cauliflower rice
- 1 cup half and half
- 1 cup shredded cheddar

Directions:

1. Heat olive oil in a pot. Season beef with salt, pepper and cook for 3 minutes.
2. Stir in onion, garlic, and tomatoes, for 5 minutes.

3. Mix in rosemary, paprika, chili and cook for 2 minutes.

4. Pour into the broth and then bring to a boil, then simmer for 25 minutes; set aside.

5. Melt butter in a pot, and cook walnuts for 3 minutes.

6. Transfer to a cutting board, chop and plate.

7. Pour cauli rice and ½ cup water into the pot and cook for 5 minutes.

8. Stir in half and half for 3 minutes. Mix in cheddar cheese, fold in walnuts. Top with stewed beef.

Nutrition Info (Per Serving): Cal 736; Net Carbs 7.8g; Fat 48g, Protein 63g

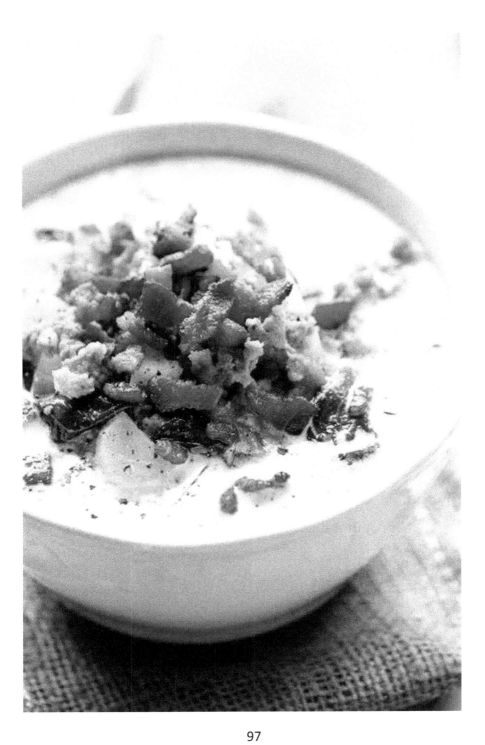

Coconut Turkey Chili

Servings: 4

Cooking Time: 30 minutes

Ingredients

- 1 pound turkey breasts, cubed
- 1 cup broccoli, chopped
- 2 shallots, sliced
- 1 (14-ounce) can of tomatoes
- 2 tbsp coconut oil
- 2 tbsp coconut cream
- 2 garlic cloves, minced
- 1 tbsp ground coriander
- 2 tbsp fresh ginger, grated
- 1 tbsp turmeric
- 1 tbsp cumin
- 2 tbsp chili powder

Directions:

1. Melt coconut oil into a pan over medium heat and stir-fry turkey, shallots, garlic, and ginger for 5 minutes. Stir in tomatoes, broccoli, turmeric, coriander, cumin, chili, salt and pepper. Pour in coconut cream and cook for 20-25 minutes. Transfer to a food processor to blend well. Serve.

Nutrition Info (Per Serving): Cal 318; Net Carbs 6.6g; Fat 18.7g; Protein 27g

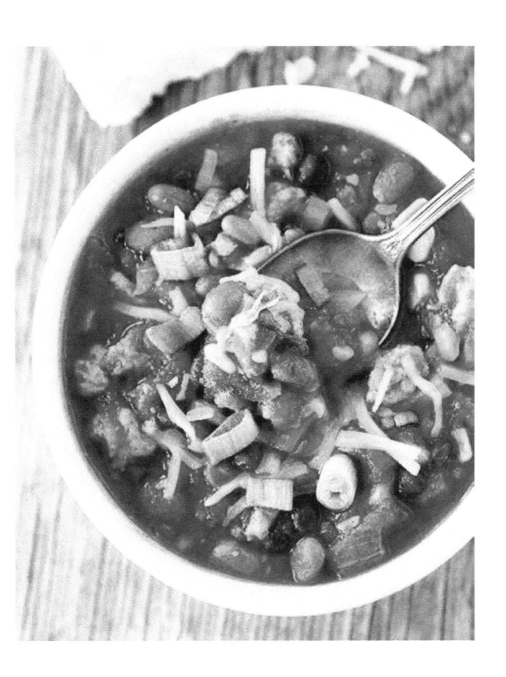

Creamed Kale with Mushrooms

Servings: 2

Cooking Time: 10 minutes

Ingredients

- ½ bunch of kale
- 3 mushrooms, sliced
- 1 ounce whipped topping
- 2 oz cream cheese
- 2 tbsp grated parmesan cheese

Seasoning:

- 1/3 tsp salt
- 1/8 tsp ground black pepper
- ¼ tsp garlic powder
- 1 ½ tbsp butter, unsalted

Directions:

1. Take a medium skillet pan, place it over medium heat, add butter and when it melts, add kale and cook for 3 minutes until tender.

2. Add remaining ingredients, stir until mixed, switch heat to the low level, and simmer for 5 to 7 minutes until mushrooms have turned tender. Serve.

Nutrition Info: 254 Calories; 23.3 g Fats; 5.5 g Protein; 3.1 g Net Carb; 0.6 g Fiber

Cremini Mushroom Stroganoff

Servings: 4

Cooking Time: 25 minutes

Ingredients

- 3 tbsp butter
- 1 white onion, chopped
- 4 cups cremini mushrooms, cubed
- 2 cups of water
- ½ cup heavy cream
- ½ cup grated Parmesan cheese
- 1 ½ tbsp dried mixed herbs
- Salt and black pepper to taste

Directions:

1. Melt the butter in a saucepan over medium heat and sauté the onion for 3 minutes until soft.

2. Stir in the mushrooms and cook until tender, about 5 minutes. Add the water, mix, and bring to boil for 10-15 minutes until the water reduces slightly. Pour in the heavy cream and Parmesan cheese. Stir to melt the cheese. Also, mix in the dried herbs. Season with salt and black pepper, simmer for 5 minutes and turn the heat off. Ladle stroganoff over a bed of spaghetti squash and serve.

Nutrition Info (Per Serving): Kcal 284, Fat 28g, Net Carbs 1,5g, Protein 8g

Creamy Zoodles

Preparation Time: 15 minutes

Cooking Time: 10 minutes

Servings: 4

Ingredients:

- 11/4 cups heavy whipping cream
- 1/4 cup mayonnaise
- Salt and ground black pepper, as required
- 30 ounces zucchini, spiralized with blade C
- 3 ounces Parmesan cheese, grated
- tablespoons fresh mint leaves
- 2 tablespoons butter, melted

Directions:

1. The heavy cream must be added to a pan then bring to a boil.
2. Lower the heat to low and cook until reduced in half.
3. Put in the pepper, mayo, and salt; cook until the mixture is warm enough. Add the zucchini noodles and gently stir to combine.
4. Stir in the Parmesan cheese.
5. Divide the zucchini noodles onto four serving plates and immediately drizzle with the melted butter.
6. Serve immediately.

Nutrition:

Calories: 241 Fat: 11.4g Fiber: 7.5g Carbohydrates: 3.1 g Protein: 5.1g

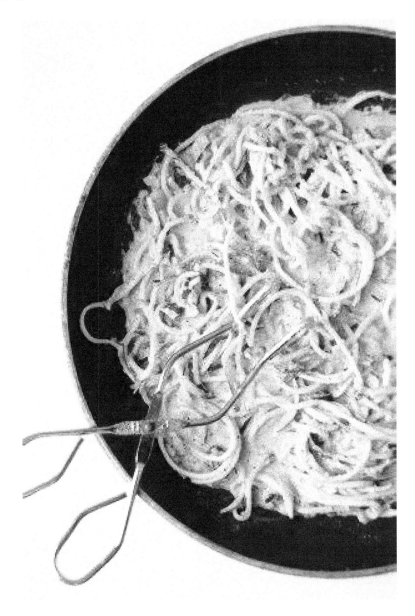

Crispy Chorizo with Cheesy Topping

Servings: 6

Cooking Time: 30 minutes

Ingredients

- 7 ounces Spanish chorizo, sliced
- 4 ounces cream cheese
- ¼ cup chopped parsley

Directions:

1. Preheat oven to 325° F. Line a baking dish with waxed paper. Bake chorizo for minutes until crispy. Remove and let cool. Arrange on a serving platter.

2. Top with cream cheese. Serve sprinkled with parsley.

Nutrition Info (Per Serving): Kcal 172, Fat: 13g, Net Carbs: 0g, Protein: 5g

Crispy Pancetta & Butternut Squash Roast

Servings: 4

Cooking Time: 30 minutes

Ingredients

- 2 butternut squash, cubed
- 1 tsp turmeric powder
- ½ tsp garlic powder
- 8 pancetta slices, chopped
- 2 tbsp olive oil
- 1 tbsp chopped cilantro

Directions:

1. Preheat oven to 425° F. In a bowl, add butternut squash, salt, pepper, turmeric, garlic powder, pancetta, and olive oil. Toss until well-coated.

2. Spread the mixture onto a greased baking sheet and roast for -15 minutes. Transfer the veggies to a bowl and garnish with cilantro to serve.

Nutrition Info (Per Serving): Cal 148; Net Carbs 6.4g; Fat 10g; Protein 6g

Crunchy Rutabaga Puffs

Servings: 4

Cooking Time: 35 minutes

Ingredients

- 1 rutabaga, peeled and diced
- 2 tbsp melted butter
- ½ oz goat cheese
- ¼ cup ground pork rinds

Directions:

1. Preheat oven to 400° F and spread rutabaga on a baking sheet. Season with salt, pepper, and drizzle with the butter. Bake until tender, minutes. Transfer to a bowl. Allow cooling and add in goat cheese. Using a fork, mash and mix the ingredients. Pour the pork rinds onto a plate. Mold 1-inch balls out of the rutabaga mixture and roll properly in the rinds while pressing gently to stick. Place on the same baking sheet and bake for 10 minutes until golden.

Nutrition Info (Per Serving): Cal 129; Net Carbs 5.9g; Fat 8g; Protein 3g

Cucumber Noodles with Avocado Sauce

Servings: 2

Cooking Time: 35 minutes

Ingredients

- 1/2 teaspoon sea salt
- 1 cucumber, spiralized
- 1 California avocado, pitted, peeled and mashed
- 1 tablespoon olive oil
- 1/2 teaspoon garlic powder
- 1/2 teaspoon paprika
- 1 tablespoon fresh lime juice

Directions:

1. Toss your cucumber with salt and let it sit for 30 minutes; discard the excess water and pat dry.

2. In a mixing bowl, thoroughly combine the avocado with olive oil, garlic powder, paprika, and lime juice.

3. Add the sauce to the cucumber noodles and serve immediately. Bon appétit!

Nutrition Info (Per Serving): 194 Calories; 17.1g Fat; 7.6g Carbs; 2.5g Protein; 4.6g Fiber

9 781803 177052